Copyright © 2020 by Eric Goldinger

All rights reserved. This book or any portion thereof may not be reproduced or used in any manner whatsoever without the express written permission of the publisher except for the use of brief quotations in a book review.

DISCLAIMER

By reading this disclaimer, you fully accept the terms of this disclaimer. If you are not in agreement with this disclaimer, please do not order or read this book. The content of this book is provided for information and educational purposes only.

The opinions expressed within this book are the personal opinions of the author. Dr. Eric Goldinger is not responsible for the accuracy, completeness, suitability, or validity of any information therein. All information is provided on an as-is basis.

Table of Contents

INTRODUCTION 6
    High Cholesterol 7
    Atherosclerosis 11
    High Cholesterol Factors 12
    Complications of High Cholesterol 14
    Causes of High Cholesterol 18
    Diagnosis of Cholesterol Levels 20
    Cholesterol Levels Measurement 21
    Cholesterol Testing for Children 24
Adoptable Lifestyle to Reduce High Cholesterol Levels 25
    1. Eat Heart-Healthy Foods 26
    2. Exercise on most days of the week and Increase your physical activity 28
    3. Quit Smoking 29
    4. Lose Weight 30
    5. Drink Alcohol Only in Moderation 30
Natural Remedies for High Cholesterol 32
    Astragalus 32
    Hawthorn 34
    Flaxseed 35
    Ginseng 36
    Artichoke Leaf Extract 36
    Green Tea 37

- Fish with omega-3 fatty acids 38
- Garlic 39
- Red Yeast Rice 39
- Coriander Seeds 40
- Plant Sterol And Stanol Supplements 41
- Psyllium Husk 41
- Fenugreek Seeds 42
- Amla 43

Home Remedy for Lower Cholesterol 44
- Optimize Your Magnesium Level 44
- Get More Vitamin C 45
- Drink Some Green Tea 45
- Add Some Vitamin K2 to Your Diet 46
- Eat Your Oatmeal 47
- Make Sure Your Thyroid is Functioning Normally 48
- Eat Some Blueberries 48
- An Apple a Day Really May Keep the Doctor Away 48
- Choose Coconut Oil for Lower Cholesterol and a Slimmer Waist 49
- Get a Little Nutty 49

High Cholesterol Diet Plans 50
- Be Selective with Your Fats 50
- Up Your Fiber Intake 52
- Eat More Whole Foods 52

How to Meal-Prep Your Week of Meals 53
    Day 1 53
    Day 2 55
    Day 3 57
    Day 4 59
    Day 5 61
    Day 6 63
    Day 7 65
    Shrimp-&-Grits-Stuffed Peppers 66
    Mediterranean Broccoli Pasta Salad 70
7-Day DASH Diet Menu 73
    Day 1 73
    Day 2 74
    Day 3 76
    Day 4 77
    Day 5 79
    Day 6 81
    Day 7 83
7-Day Mediterranean Meal Plan 85
    Day 1 85
    Day 2 86
    Day 3 87
    Day 4 89

Day 5 90
Day 6 91
Day 7 93

INTRODUCTION

The health sector throughout the world has recently gain attraction, diverse symptoms, aliments and so on sprung up at intervals due to human's negligence to the content of what we eat.

When was the last time you visited your doctor for a routine check-up? Well, I just reminded you right? Oh! The cruel reality is that when it comes to our health, most of the time we are lazy or nonchalant. Because of the modern lifestyle we're engaged in, we're always rushing or chasing a lot of things while at the same time neglecting to take proper care of ourselves.

High cholesterol is often a silent killer not accompanied by visible symptoms. High cholesterol puts you at risk for life-threatening diseases such as heart attacks and strokes. If you have been diagnosed with high cholesterol or have the potential to become a victim of various family histories, one thing is certain: to win the battle against cholesterol and live a long and happy life, you need information to prepare yourself and make changes to your lifestyle. In this book, put together to help you achieve those goals.

The book will help you gain a comprehensive understanding of high cholesterol, its risk factors, its causes and related diseases. Medical treatment for high cholesterol may not fix or provide a long-term solution to the actual cause of your illness. This book will help you learn more about positive lifestyle changes, healthy diet plans, and natural remedies that will allow you to take control of your health and start lowering your cholesterol well. It's always better and easy to prevent diseases than curing a disease.

High Cholesterol

People are getting more confused about fat and cholesterol and the majority find them the same.

Fat varies significantly from cholesterol; they are two different subgroups of a broad category called lipids.

Cholesterol is good and poor respectively. It is an essential material for the body, at normal levels. If blood concentrations get too high, however, it becomes a silent danger which puts people at risk of heart attack.

Cholesterol is present in every cell of the body and has important natural roles in food digestion, hormone production, and vitamin D generation. It is created by the body but it is also ingested in food by people. In appearance it is waxy and fat-like.

High cholesterol is one of the major risk factors for heart disease. It increases your chance of developing heart disease and having a heart attack. It can also raise your risk of stroke. This plaque, which consists of cholesterol fatty deposits, gradually narrows the lumen of the arteries and impedes oxygen and nutrient supply to the heart.

Cholesterol is a fatty substance in the blood. There are two types of cholesterol. A correct balance between the two is needed for good health.

High-density lipoprotein (HDL) or "good" cholesterol helps remove excess cholesterol from the body. Low-density lipoprotein (LDL) or "bad" cholesterol can cause cholesterol to build up in the arteries.

Low HDL or high LDL cholesterol increases the risk of coronary heart disease. LDL cholesterol forms a substance called plaque in the arteries of the heart. Over time, this plaque can build up, form a clot, and block the arteries of the heart. This may result in chest pain or a heart attack.

High cholesterol usually means too much LDL. There are no symptoms, so many people are unaware they have it. Having high cholesterol can double the risk of heart disease, compared with normal levels.

Triglycerides are another type of fat in your blood. When you eat more calories than your body can use, it turns the extra calories into triglycerides.

Your ideal cholesterol level will depend on your risk for heart disease.

- Total cholesterol level – less than 200 is best, but it depends on your HDL and LDL levels.
- LDL cholesterol levels – less than 130 is best, but this depends on your risk for heart disease.
- HDL cholesterol levels – 60 or higher reduces your risk for heart disease.
- Triglycerides – less than 150 milligrams per deciliter (mg/dl) is best.

Older people have a greater chance for having increased levels of cholesterol likewise men have a greater chance of developing high cholesterol than women.

Atherosclerosis

Excess cholesterol can be laid down in the walls of your arteries. Fatty areas known as plaques can form, and these become harder with time, making the arteries stiffer and narrower.

- **Narrowed Arteries**

When the arteries become narrower, it's harder for blood to flow through them. This puts a strain on your heart because it has to work harder to pump blood around your body. Eventually, the heart can become weak and can't work as well as it should.

- **Blood Clots**

Blood clots can form over the fatty, hardened parts of the arteries. The blood clots can block the artery completely, cutting off the blood flow. Bits of the blood clots can break away and become lodged in an artery or vein in another part of the body, which can cause a heart attack or stroke.

High Cholesterol Factors

Factors that can increase your risk of bad cholesterol include:

- Poor diet. You can increase the cholesterol level by consuming saturated fat contained in animal products and trans fats contained in some commercially baked cookies and crackers and microwave popcorn. Your cholesterol will also be increased by foods that are high in cholesterol, such as red meat and full-fat dairy products.

- Obesity. Having a body mass index (BMI) of 30 or greater puts you at risk of high cholesterol.
- Lack of exercise. Exercise helps boost the HDL or "healthy" cholesterol in your body while increasing the size of the particles that make up the LDL, or "bad" cholesterol, making it less harmful.
- Smoking. Cigarette smoking damages the walls of your blood vessels, making them more prone to accumulate fatty deposits. Smoking might also lower your level of HDL, or "good," cholesterol.
- Age. As the chemistry of the body changes with the age, the risk of high cholesterol is increasing. Your liver, for example, becomes less able to remove LDL cholesterol as you age.
- Diabetes. High blood sugar leads to higher cholesterol levels called very-low-density

lipoprotein (VLDL) and lower HDL cholesterol levels. High sugar in the blood also affects the lining of the arteries.

Complications of High Cholesterol

If your arteries become clogged up with blood fats, your blood can't flow around your body easily. This can lead to a number of diseases of the heart and blood vessels.

These diseases are known together as cardiovascular disease – cardio refers to the heart, and vascular refers to the blood vessels.

Coronary Heart Disease (Coronary Artery Disease)

This is where the arteries have become clogged up and stiff with atherosclerosis. The blood can't flow around the body and back to the heart easily, and blood clots can form. This can lead to chest pain, heart failure, heart attacks and strokes.

Angina (Chest Pain)

This is a dull, heavy or tight pain in the chest which can spread to the left arm, neck, jaw or back. It happens when the arteries leading to the heart have become narrowed and the heart doesn't get enough oxygen. The pain can be brought on by exercise or activity, as the heart needs more oxygen during physical activity.

A Heart Attack

This is a medical emergency. It happens when an artery leading to the heart becomes completely blocked, often by a blood clot, cutting off the blood supply. Part of the heart muscle quickly dies, but if it's treated very early the blockage can be removed.

The signs of a heart attack include:

- A crushing pain in the chest
- Sweating
- Shortness of breath

- Feeling or being sick
- Feeling weak or faint

Heart Failure

This is not the same as a heart attack. Heart failure usually happens when the arteries are clogged up and the heart has to work too hard to force blood around the body. To start with, the heart muscle gets bigger to cope with the extra effort, but eventually it becomes too weak and can't push blood around your body.

It doesn't mean your heart is about to stop working but it can cause serious problems, including breathing problems because the blood can't flow around your lungs easily.

Stroke

This is a medical emergency. It happens when an artery in or leading to the brain becomes blocked, cutting off the blood supply. Part of the brain dies which can cause disabilities. Getting treatment straight away can lower the risk of long-term problems.

The signs include:

- The face droops on one side
- Slurred speech or being unable to talk or smile
- Weakness in the arms or not being able to lift them.

Mini Strokes (TIAs)

Blocked blood vessels can also cause mini strokes known as TIAs (transient ischaemic attack). These are temporary, and the signs of a stroke pass within 24 hours, usually after a few minutes. Mini strokes are a warning sign that you could have a full stroke.

See your doctor straight away if you think you have had a TIA so that you can get treatment and support to prevent a stroke.

Peripheral Arterial Disease (PAD)

This is when one or more of the arteries leading to the legs and feet become blocked or narrowed, so not enough blood can reach them. This can make your feet feel cold and painful, especially when walking. It can be hard to walk, and the worst-case scenario is that the foot needs to be amputated.

Vascular Dementia

There are different types of dementia, and vascular dementia is the second most common type. It can cause problems with memory, thinking and talking. It's caused by problems with the blood supply to the brain – either by a stroke or mini strokes, or because the blood vessels in the brain have become too narrow.

Causes of High Cholesterol

High cholesterol is a major risk factor for heart disease and a reason for heart attacks.

A build-up of cholesterol is part of a cycle called atherosclerosis, which narrows arteries. Plaques form in atherosclerosis, which cause blood flow restriction.

Reducing the dietary fat intake helps control cholesterol levels. Especially limiting foods which contain:

- Cholesterol: This is present in animal foods, meat, and cheese.
- Saturated fat: This occurs in some meats, dairy products, chocolate, baked goods, deep-fried, and processed foods.
- Trans fats: This occurs in some fried and processed foods.

Excess weight or obesity can also lead to higher blood LDL levels. Genetic factors can contribute to high cholesterol. People with the inherited condition familial hypercholesterolemia have very high LDL levels.

Other conditions that can lead to high cholesterol levels include:

- Diabetes
- Liver or kidney disease
- Polycystic ovary syndrome
- Pregnancy and other conditions that increase levels of female hormones
- Underactive thyroid gland
- Drugs that increase LDL cholesterol and decrease HDL cholesterol, such as progestin, anabolic steroids, and corticosteroids

Diagnosis of Cholesterol Levels

A blood test to check cholesterol levels called a lipid panel or lipid profile typically reports:

- Total cholesterol
- LDL cholesterol
- HDL cholesterol
- Triglycerides a type of fat in the blood

Do not eat or drink something (other than water) for nine to 12 hours before taking the blood sample, for the most precise measurements.

Cholesterol Levels Measurement

In the United States, cholesterol levels are measured in milligrams (mg) of cholesterol per deciliter (dL) of blood. In Canada and many European countries, cholesterol levels are measured in millimoles per liter (mmol/L). To interpret your test results, use these general guidelines.

Total cholesterol (U.S. and some other countries)	Total cholesterol* (Canada and most of Europe)	Results
Below 200 mg/dL	Below 5.2 mmol/L	Desirable
200-239 mg/dL	5.2-6.2 mmol/L	Borderline high
240 mg/dL and above	Above 6.2 mmol/L	High

*Canadian and European guidelines differ slightly from U.S. guidelines. These conversions are based on U.S. guidelines.

LDL cholesterol (U.S. and some other countries)	LDL cholesterol* (Canada and most of Europe)	Results
Below 70 mg/dL	Below 1.8 mmol/L	Best for people who have heart disease or diabetes.
Below 100 mg/dL	Below 2.6 mmol/L	Optimal for people at risk of heart disease.
100-129 mg/dL	2.6-3.3 mmol/L	Near optimal if there is no heart disease. High if there is heart disease.
130-159 mg/dL	3.4-4.1 mmol/L	Borderline high if there is no heart disease. High if there is heart disease.
160-189 mg/dL	4.1-4.9 mmol/L	High if there is no heart disease. Very high if there is heart disease.
190 mg/dL and above	Above 4.9 mmol/L	Very high

*Canadian and European guidelines differ slightly from U.S. guidelines. These conversions are based on U.S. guidelines.

HDL cholesterol (U.S. and some other countries)	HDL cholesterol*(Canada and most of Europe)	Results
Below 40 mg/dL, men Below 50 mg/dL, women	Below 1 mmol/L Below 1.3 mmol/L	Poor
40-59 mg/dL, men 50-59 mg.dL, women	1-1.5 mmol/L 1.3-1.5 mmol/L	Better
60 mg/dL and above	Above 1.5 mmol/L	Best

Triglycerides (U.S. and some other countries)	Triglycerides* (Canada and most of Europe)	Results
Below 150 mg/dL	Below 1.7 mmol/L	Desirable
150-199 mg/dL	1.7-2.2 mmol/L	Borderline High
200-499 mg/dL	2.3-5.6 mmol/L	High
500 mg/dL and above	Above 5.6 mmol/L	Very high

*Canadian and European guidelines differ slightly from U.S. guidelines. These conversions are based on U.S. guidelines.

Cholesterol Testing for Children

You probably know that you need to get your blood lipids, or cholesterol, checked regularly as a way to understand your risk for cardiovascular disease. But you might wonder why your 10 year old needs to have her cholesterol checked. With increasing rates of diabetes, obesity and other risk factors for cardiovascular disease, monitoring blood lipid levels is one way we can help to keep your child healthy.

Current guidelines from the National Heart, Lung, and Blood Institute recommend that children aged 9 to 11 years of age and young adults 17 to 21 years of age be screened for high cholesterol, regardless of risk factors.

In fact, if your child has elevated lipids in a previous test or risk factors for cardiovascular disease, your doctor may want to test their cholesterol levels earlier or more frequently.

If your child's cholesterol levels are high or borderline, you are encouraged to work with your doctor to manage them through diet and exercise modifications. However, if diet and exercise do not help, or levels are extremely high, your child should see a pediatric cardiologist.

Adoptable Lifestyle to Reduce High Cholesterol Levels

Heart diseases in the United States of America are rampant; cholesterol lowering has thus become a major problem attracting attention. While several other factors contribute to hearing impairment, high cholesterol is a significant risk factor. Going natural is the safest way to reduce high cholesterol other than pharmaceutical drugs.

Although cholesterol drugs can return the LDL levels to their normal range, most drugs only target the symptoms of the condition and are not designed to address the actual source of high cholesterol, or provide a long-term solution. Healthy lifestyle changes cannot only improve your cholesterol levels, but your overall health as well. You will not only be stopping the plaque from forming in your arteries, but you will be keeping other conditions like high blood pressure, diabetes, and obesity, from becoming a part of your life. If bad habits are contributing to your cholesterol condition, it is time to take action and make changes. In case you have no idea where to start, here are the steps to follow.

1. Eat Heart-Healthy Foods

A few changes in your diet can reduce cholesterol and improve your heart health:

- Reduce saturated fats. Saturated fats, found primarily in red meat and full-fat dairy products, raise your total cholesterol. Decreasing your consumption of saturated fats can reduce your low-density lipoprotein (LDL) cholesterol the "bad" cholesterol.

- Eliminate trans fats. Trans fats, sometimes listed on food labels as "partially hydrogenated vegetable oil," are often used in margarines and store-bought cookies, crackers and cakes. Trans fats raise overall cholesterol levels. The Food and Drug Administration has banned the use of partially hydrogenated vegetable oils by Jan. 1, 2021.
- Eat foods rich in omega-3 fatty acids. Omega-3 fatty acids don't affect LDL cholesterol. But they have other heart-healthy benefits, including reducing blood pressure. Foods with omega-3 fatty acids include salmon, mackerel, herring, walnuts and flaxseeds.
- Increase soluble fiber. Soluble fiber can reduce the absorption of cholesterol into your bloodstream. Soluble fiber is found in

such foods as oatmeal, kidney beans, Brussels sprouts, apples and pears.
- Add whey protein. Whey protein, which is found in dairy products, may account for many of the health benefits attributed to dairy. Studies have shown that whey protein given as a supplement lowers both LDL cholesterol and total cholesterol as well as blood pressure.

2. Exercise on most days of the week and Increase your physical activity

Exercise can improve cholesterol. Moderate physical activity can help raise high-density lipoprotein (HDL) cholesterol, the "good" cholesterol. With your doctor's OK, work up to at least 30 minutes of exercise five times a week or vigorous aerobic activity for 20 minutes three times a week.

Adding physical activity, even in short intervals several times a day can help you begin to lose weight. Consider:

- Taking a brisk daily walk during your lunch hour
- Riding your bike to work
- Playing a favorite sport

To stay motivated, consider finding an exercise buddy or joining an exercise group.

3. Quit Smoking

Quitting smoking improves your HDL cholesterol level. The benefits occur quickly:

- Within 20 minutes of quitting, your blood pressure and heart rate recover from the cigarette-induced spike
- Within three months of quitting, your blood circulation and lung function begin to improve

- Within a year of quitting, your risk of heart disease is half that of a smoker

4. Lose Weight

Carrying even a few extra pounds contributes to high cholesterol. Small changes add up. If you drink sugary beverages, switch to tap water. Snack on air-popped popcorn or pretzels but keep track of the calories. If you crave something sweet, try sherbet or candies with little or no fat, such as jelly beans.

Look for ways to incorporate more activity into your daily routine, such as using the stairs instead of taking the elevator or parking farther from your office. Take walks during breaks at work. Try to increase standing activities, such as cooking or doing yardwork.

5. Drink Alcohol Only in Moderation

Moderate use of alcohol has been linked with higher levels of HDL cholesterol but the benefits aren't strong enough to recommend alcohol for anyone who doesn't already drink.

If you drink alcohol, do so in moderation. For healthy adults, that means up to one drink a day for women of all ages and men older than age 65, and up to two drinks a day for men age 65 and younger.

Too much alcohol can lead to serious health problems, including high blood pressure, heart failure and strokes.

Natural Remedies for High Cholesterol

Natural or complementary heart disease therapies also aim at reducing cholesterol levels, decreasing blood pressure and improving heart safety. Research on these treatments is usually minimal, compared to traditional medical treatments.

Few natural products have been clinically proven to reduce cholesterol. Before you try any alternative treatments, check with your doctor to determine if they're safe for you. The ingredients in some alternative therapies can interfere with certain medications or have harmful side effects.

Astragalus

Astragalus is a herb used in traditional Chinese medicine to strengthen the immune system. It has anti-inflammatory and antibacterial properties. It's considered to be an "adaptogen." This means it's believed to protect the body against various stresses. It is also used as a "Qi tonifier" in the oriental system of medicine. The root is the only part of the plant used medicinally and is usually harvested from 4-year old plants.

Proponents:

- Boosts the Immune system
- Helps combat infections
- Has antioxidant and anti-inflammatory effects
- Protects the kidneys and heart
- May have anticancer effects

Skeptics:

- Interacts with immunosuppressant
- May not be suitable for autoimmune conditions
- People report headaches and insomnia from higher doses
- Most conditions require intravenous application

Potentially Active Chemical Constituents

Polysaccharides are the most important functional constituents in Astragalus and responsible for the antimicrobial, antiviral and anti-inflammatory capabilities of this herb.

It also has several saponins, called Astragalosides (I to X) which are known for their ability to lower cholesterol and boost the immune system.

Astragalus also contains flavonoids which demonstrate antioxidant properties and help prevent heart disease and immunodeficiency. Other elements are amino acids, folic acid, etc., and minerals such as selenium, zinc, and copper.

Hawthorn

The hawthorn berry plant has been a part of ancient medicine across the world, including Europe, the Americas, and China. Both the berry and leaves are edible, and people can use the entire plant for its health benefits. Hawthorn has antioxidant properties similar to astragalus, which help to support the functioning of the cardiovascular system. Research suggests that hawthorn can support healthy levels of total cholesterol, LDL cholesterol, and triglycerides (these are fats in the blood – your doctor measures your level of triglycerides when they perform a cholesterol blood test).

Flaxseed

Though not an herb, flaxseed is one of those wonder foods that are touted to help against many serious conditions, including heart disease. Flaxseed may support healthy cholesterol levels and overall heart health. You can find flaxseed at the grocery store in ground form or alongside many other herbs in the supplement aisle.

Ginseng

Ginseng is an herb that has been used in Asian medicine for centuries, typically mixed with other herbs. Folk medicine used ginseng to treat a variety of ailments and support heart health. These days, ginseng root is sold in capsules and many popular products green teas, coffees, and even energy drinks. Some studies show that ginseng may support healthy levels of "bad" LDL cholesterol and "good" HDL cholesterol.

Artichoke Leaf Extract

Like ginseng, artichoke leaf extract has long been used throughout history in medicine, and one of its most popular uses is as an aid in supporting healthy cholesterol. In several clinical trials, artichoke leaf extract has shown an impact on supporting healthy levels of "bad" LDL and total cholesterol. [HB1] Researchers have struggled to replicate the most promising numbers seen in studies, but the findings are encouraging rtichoke leaf extract may be one of the best herbs to support healthy levels of cholesterol that's out there on the market.

Green Tea

The most consumed liquid after water, green tea is a rich source of polyphenols. These compounds provide immense health benefits to the human body. Green tea has the highest concentration of polyphenols associated with not only lowering LDL Cholesterol but also increasing HDL Cholesterol. A population based study showed that men who drank green tea had lower cholesterol levels as compared to those who didn't. Studies have indicated that the polyphenols of tea may block cholesterol absorption in the intestines and also help get rid of it. 2-3 cups of green tea is all you need.

Fish with omega-3 fatty acids

Omega-3 fatty acids are also found in fish and fish oils. Salmon, tuna, lake trout, herring, sardines, and other fatty fish are especially rich sources. It has long believed that omega-3 fatty acids in fish help reduce the risk of dying from heart disease. More recent studies suggest that other nutrients in fish, or a combination of those nutrients and omega-3 fatty acids, may help protect your heart. Eating one or two servings of fatty fish per week may lower your chances of dying from a heart attack.

If you have heart disease, you may also benefit from taking omega-3 fatty acid supplements or eating other foods rich in omega-3 fatty acids. For example, walnuts, canola oil, and soybeans are good sources. However, the Mayo Clinic notes that the evidence is stronger for the benefits of eating fish with omega-3 fatty acids than taking supplements or eating other foods.

Garlic

Garlic is an edible bulb that's been used as a cooking ingredient and medicine for thousands of years. It can be eaten raw or cooked. It's also available in supplement form, as a capsule or tablet.

Garlic help lower your blood pressure, reduce your blood cholesterol levels, and slow the progress of atherosclerosis. However, as with many alternative therapies, studies have yielded mixed results. For example, some studies have found that taking garlic for one to three months helps lower blood cholesterol levels. However, an NCCIH-funded study on the safety and effectiveness of three garlic preparations found no long-term effect on blood cholesterol.

Red Yeast Rice

Red yeast rice is a traditional Chinese medicine and cooking ingredient. It's made by culturing red rice with yeast.

Some red yeast rice products contain substantial quantities of monacolin K, This substance is chemically identical to the active ingredient in the cholesterol-lowering drug lovastatin. Red yeast rice products that contain this substance help lower your blood cholesterol levels.

Other red yeast rice products contain little to no monacolin K, some also contain a contaminant called citrinin. This contaminant can cause kidney failure. In many cases, there's no way for you to know which products contain monacolin K or citrinin. Therefore, it's hard to tell which products will be effective or safe.

Coriander Seeds

The humble Dhaniya seeds have been used in Ayurveda for a number of ailments. Among the long list, lowering bad cholesterol is one of them.Coriander seeds have numerous key vitamins like folic acid, vitamin A and beta-carotene, and most importantly, vitamin C.

Plant Sterol And Stanol Supplements

Plant sterols and stanols are substances found in many fruits, vegetables, nuts, seeds, grains, and other plants. Some processed foods are also fortified with plant sterols or stanols. For example, you may find fortified margarines, orange juice, or yogurt products.

Research suggests that plant sterols and stanols may help lower your risk of heart disease. They help prevent your small intestine from absorbing cholesterol. This can lower "bad" LDL cholesterol levels in your blood.

Psyllium Husk

In 1998, the US FDA approved of a health claim on Psyllium –"3 to 12 grams of soluble fiber from psyllium seed husk when included as part of a diet low in saturated fat and cholesterol, may reduce the risk of heart disease". Psyllium husk comes from the crushed seeds of the Plantago Ovata plant and is a rich source of soluble fibre. There are innumerable studies to substantiate the benefits of soluble fibre in lowering LDL cholesterol. Adding 1-2 teaspoons of psyllium husk to our daily meals contributes the soluble fibre needed for keeping our cholesterol under check.

Fenugreek Seeds

Methi seeds, as they are known to us, have been used as a popular culinary spice, flavouring agent and a medicinal plant since time immemorial. Methi seeds are rich in Vitamin E and possess antidiabetic, anti-inflammatory, and antioxidant properties. Saponins found in fenugreek help remove cholesterol from the body and its fibre helps reduce the synthesis in the liver. 1/2 to 1 teaspoon of fenugreek seeds daily is recommended.

Amla

It is one of the richest sources of Vitamin C and phenolic compounds in addition to minerals and amino acids. The fruit of amla has been used in Ayurveda as a rasayan for the treatment of various diseases. A study published in the Indian Journal of Pharmacology, compared the effect of cholesterol lowering drugs against amla. In addition to reducing cholesterol, amla was found to provide the additional benefit of protection against atherosclerosis and CAD. Daily intake of amla not only reduces bad cholesterol levels but also reduces the damage due to oxidation. One to two amla fruits can be consumed daily.

These foods should be consumed in their natural form as a part of a healthy lifestyle to achieve your health goals. Medication to lower cholesterol should not be taken or discontinued without the doctor's orders.

Home Remedy for Lower Cholesterol

Optimize Your Magnesium Level

Magnesium acts as a natural statin, limiting cholesterol production so that it covers necessary functions but is not produced in excess. Foods that are high in magnesium include: kelp, wheat bran, wheat germ, almonds, cashews, molasses, brewer's yeast, buckwheat, Brazil nuts, dulse, filberts, peanuts, wheat grain, millet, pecans, English walnuts, rye, tofu and dark chocolate.

Many wild plants are also high in magnesium, such as burdock root, dandelion, chickweed and nettle. It may be difficult for people to get enough magnesium through diet, so applying magnesium oil topically can also be helpful.

Get More Vitamin C

As an antioxidant, vitamin C helps to reduce inflammation. Some good sources of vitamin C include:

- Citrus fruits such as oranges, grapefruit, lemons and limes
- Kiwi
- Papaya
- Strawberries
- Pineapple
- Cantaloupe
- Sweet bell peppers – green or red
- Cruciferous vegetables such as cabbage, cauliflower, broccoli and kale
- Sweet potatoes

Drink Some Green Tea

Catechin, a major constituent of green tea, has been shown to reduce oxidized (damaged) low-density lipoprotein.

Add Some Vitamin K2 to Your Diet

K2 can lower serum cholesterol, more importantly; K2 reduces atherosclerois, i.e. plaque accumulation in the arteries. This plaque is the deposits of calcium, fatty substances and scar tissue that together cause "hardening of the arteries". With plaque buildup, the arteries either clog up and reduce or stop blood flow entirely, or get fragile and have a blowout. Vitamin K2 is not the same as vitamin K1, which is abundant in leafy greens and great for bone building.

Vitamin K2 works in concert with calcium and vitamin D, making sure the calcium gets where it's needed in your bones, not your muscles and arteries. In addition, vitamin K2 can remove calcium buildup in the arteries after it has formed and help restore arterial flexibility. The best source of vitamin K2 is natto, a fermented soybean concoction with a stringy, slimy texture. Other sources of vitamin K2 include goose liver pate, hard cheeses (such as gouda), soft cheeses (such as Brie), egg yolk, butter and chicken liver. Most people in the US are low in vitamin K2, although regular cheese eaters tend to far better than the general population. You can also buy a K2 supplement made from natto.

Eat Your Oatmeal

As the much publicized commercials for popular cereal brands note, the soluble fiber in oats helps to lower total and LDL cholesterol levels. Go ahead and enjoy a nice warn bowl of oatmeal (soak overnight for quick morning cooking and easier digestion) or sneak some oatmeal into your snacking with fun recipes.

Make Sure Your Thyroid is Functioning Normally

Hypothyroidism (under active thyroid) often correlates with high cholesterol levels. Talk to your health care provider about checking your thyroid. Improving thyroid function may help to naturally reduce cholesterol levels.

Eat Some Blueberries

Blueberry intake acutely improves vascular function in healthy men in a time- and dose-dependent manner. Blueberries are high in anti-oxidants, which reduce inflammation.

An Apple a Day Really May Keep the Doctor Away

My grandmother Alice always loved to say, "An apple a day keeps the doctor away". It turns out she was probably right. A 2011 study by researchers from Florida State University found that older women who ate apples every day reduced LDL cholesterol levels by 23% within six months and increased HDL cholesterol levels by 4%. The apple eating women also lost an average of 3.3 pounds.

Choose Coconut Oil for Lower Cholesterol and a Slimmer Waist

In a 2011 study, woman consuming about 2 tablespoons of coconut oil per day experienced increased levels of HDL, decreased LDL/HDL ratio and reduced waist circumferences. For a sweet treat that includes coconut oil, cocoa (for magnesium) and walnuts.

Get a Little Nutty

Walnuts, like fish oil, are also high in omega-3 fatty acids. Nuts are also high in magnesium. In an unrelated note, getting a little silly to reduce stress is also very good for reducing inflammation and improving overall health.

High Cholesterol Diet Plans

High cholesterol levels are often treated with a combination of prescribed medication and changes in diet and lifestyle. Depending on your individual needs, these healthy eating tips can help lower your cholesterol to a safe level with or without taking medication. When you pair these simple high cholesterol diet tips with other safe lifestyle practices, such as exercising daily, not smoking, and consuming less alcohol, you'll see your health improving, and cholesterol levels fall even faster to a healthier range.

Be Selective with Your Fats

Though it sounds backward, foods high in dietary cholesterol (such as shrimp and eggs) don't actually seem to raise our body's cholesterol levels. To lower your cholesterol, limit foods with saturated fats (like red meat, processed meats such as hot dogs and sausage, and cheese and other high-fat dairy items) and instead, go for leaner white meat (like chicken and turkey) and plant-based protein options (like tofu and beans), and switch over to low-fat dairy products. Additionally, you'll want to include more heart-healthy fats from foods like salmon, avocados, olive oil, nuts and seeds, which help to improve cholesterol levels.

A measure that can have an even greater effect on lowering cholesterol levels is the removal of foods produced from hydrogenated fats and partially hydrogenated fats (also known as trans fats), which are highly refined fats (commonly found in shelf-stable baked foods and processed peanut butter) associated with increased risk of heart disease, type 2 diabetes and Alzheimer's disease. As of January 2020, the FDA barred food producers from adding trans fats, but still review the ingredient lists and avoid products identified with hydrogenated or partially hydrogenated fats.

Up Your Fiber Intake

Increasing your intake of fibre can help reduce your cholesterol. We do this for you in the meal plan below-the plan's every day contains about 30 grams of fiber, which is the daily amount recommended. Most of us know that fiber plays an important role in keeping our digestive processes going along, but cholesterol can also be lowered by binding to the fat in our gut, which prevents our body from consuming it. Fruits and vegetables, whole grains (like oatmeal and brown rice), as well as beans and lentils are strong sources of fibre.

Eat More Whole Foods

When consuming more whole foods , such as fruits, vegetables , whole grains, beans and lentils, nuts and seeds and other healthy fats, there would be less space for non-healthy foods that can either increase cholesterol levels or lead to other heart-related issues. Foods (ad drinks) containing excess sodium and added sugars can lead to increased blood pressure and weight gain, both precursors of heart disease. When your diet consists mostly of nutritious whole foods, it will have less effect when you're really missing a juicy steak or the doughnut.

How to Meal-Prep Your Week of Meals

Set yourself up for success this week by getting some meal prep done in advance.

- Prepare Meal-Prep Turkey Cobb Salad to have for lunch on Days 2 through 5
- Make the Citrus Vinaigrette to have throughout the week.
- Bake a batch of the Maple Granola to have throughout the week.

Day 1

Breakfast (255 calories)

- 1 serving Strawberry-Pineapple Smoothie

A.M. Snack (59 calories)

- 1 medium peach

Lunch (325 calories)

- 1 serving Veggie & Hummus Sandwich

P.M. Snack (105 calories)

- 8 walnut halves

Dinner (458 calories)

- 1 serving Greek Grilled Salmon Kebabs with Tzatziki & Green Beans

- 1 serving Persian Cucumber & Tomato Salad with Preserved Lemon

Daily Totals: 1,201 calories, 59 g protein, 129 g carbohydrates, 30 g fiber, 56 g fat, 8 g saturated fat, 1,345 mg sodium

To make it 1,500 calories: Add ¼ cup dry roasted unsalted almonds to A.M. snack and 1 pear to lunch.

To make it 2,000 calories: Add 1 slice whole-wheat toast with 1½ Tbsp. almond butter to breakfast, ¼ cup unsalted dry-roasted almonds to A.M. snack and 1 banana to lunch, increase walnut halves to ¼ cup at P.M. snack and add a 2-oz. slice of whole-wheat baguette to dinner.

Day 2

Breakfast (274 calories)

- 1 cup nonfat Greek yogurt
- ½ cup blackberries
- ¼ cup Maple Granola

A.M. Snack (64 calories)

- 1 cup raspberries

Lunch (305 calories)

- 1 serving Meal-Prep Turkey Cobb Salad

- 1 plum

P.M. Snack (159 calories)

- 2/3 cup blueberries

- 2 Tbsp. unsalted dry-roasted almonds

Dinner (403 calories)

- 1 serving Vegetarian Lo Mein with Shiitakes, Carrots & Bean Sprouts

- 2 cups mixed greens

- 1 Tbsp. Citrus Vinaigrette

Daily Totals: 1,205 calories, 59 g protein, 120 g carbohydrates, 29 g fiber, 58 g fat, 9 g saturated fat, 1,266 mg sodium

To make it 1,500 calories: Increase Maple Granola to 1/3 cup at breakfast, add ½ an avocado to lunch and increase almonds to ¼ cup in the P.M. snack.

To make it 2,000 calories: Increase Maple Granola to 1/3 cup and add 1 slice whole-wheat toast with 1½ Tbsp. almond butter to breakfast, add ¼ cup unsalted dry-roasted almonds to A.M. snack, add 1 banana and ½ an avocado to lunch, and increase almonds to ¼ cup at P.M. snack.

Meal-Prep Tip: Prepare 1 serving of Date & Pine Nut Overnight Oatmeal to have for breakfast tomorrow.

Day 3

Breakfast (281 calories)

- 1 serving Date & Pine Nut Overnight Oatmeal

A.M. Snack (101 calories)

- 1 medium pear

Lunch (305 calories)

- 1 serving Meal-Prep Turkey Cobb Salad

- 1 plum

P.M. Snack (31 calories)

- ½ cup blackberries

Dinner (464 calories)

- 1 serving Sheet-Pan Chicken Fajita Bowls

- 1 serving Jason Mraz's Guacamole

Daily Totals: 1,183 calories, 68 g protein, 127 g carbohydrates, 32 g fiber, 52 g fat, 9 g saturated fat, 1,307 mg sodium

To make it 1,500 calories: Add ½ an avocado to lunch and 10 walnut halves to P.M. snack.

To make it 2,000 calories: Add 1 cup plain nonfat Greek yogurt to breakfast, add ¼ cup unsalted dry-roasted almonds to A.M. snack, add 1 banana and ½ an avocado to lunch, add 6 walnut halves to P.M. snack, and add 1 oz. corn tortilla chips to dinner.

Day 4

Breakfast (274 calories)

- 1 cup nonfat plain Greek yogurt

- ½ cup blackberries

- ¼ cup Maple Granola

A.M. Snack (59 calories)

- 1 peach

Lunch (305 calories)

- 1 serving Meal-Prep Turkey Cobb Salad

- 1 plum

P.M. Snack (64 calories)

- 1 cup raspberries

Dinner (500 calories)

- 1 serving Salsa-Black Bean Burgers

- 1 serving Grilled Sweet Potato Wedges

Daily Totals: 1,201 calories, 57 g protein, 135 g carbohydrates, 32 g fiber, 52 g fat, 9 g saturated fat, 1,389 mg sodium

To make it 1,500 calories: Increase Maple Granola to 1/3 cup at breakfast, add 8 walnut halves to A.M. snack and add ½ an avocado to lunch.

To make it 2,000 calories: Add 1 slice whole-wheat toast and 1½ Tbsp. almond butter to breakfast, add ¼ cup unsalted dry-roasted almonds to A.M. snack, add 1 banana and ½ an avocado to lunch, and add 1 5-oz. container nonfat plain Greek yogurt to P.M. snack.

Meal-Prep Tip: Prepare 1 serving of Date & Pine Nut Overnight Oatmeal to have for breakfast tomorrow.

Day 5

Breakfast (281 calories)

- 1 serving Date & Pine Nut Overnight Oatmeal

A.M. Snack (41 calories)

- 2/3 cup blackberries

Lunch (305 calories)

- 1 serving Meal-Prep Turkey Cobb Salad
- 1 plum

P.M. Snack (126 calories)

- 2/3 cup raspberries
- 1 5-oz. container nonfat plain Greek yogurt

Dinner (459 calories)

- 1 serving Turkish Seared Tuna with Bulgur & Chickpea Salad

Daily Totals: 1,213 calories, 74 g protein, 130 g carbohydrates, 28 g fiber, 48 g fat, 9 g saturated fat, 1,257 mg sodium

To make it 1,500 calories: Add ½ an avocado to lunch and add ¼ cup Maple Granola to P.M. snack.

To make it 2,000 calories: Add 1 cup nonfat plain Greek yogurt to breakfast, ¼ cup unsalted dry-roasted almonds to A.M. snack, ½ an avocado and 1 banana to lunch, and 1 serving Balsamic & Parmesan Roasted Broccoli to dinner.

Day 6

Breakfast (274 calories)

- 1 cup nonfat plain Greek yogurt
- ½ cup blackberries
- ¼ cup Maple Granola

A.M. Snack (83 calories)

- 1 plum
- 4 walnut halves

Lunch (304 calories)

- 1 serving Green Goddess Salad with Chickpeas

P.M. Snack (101 calories)

- 1 medium pear

Dinner (439 calories)

- 1 serving BBQ Chicken Tacos with Red Cabbage Slaw

- 2 cups mixed greens

- 1 Tbsp. Citrus Vinaigrette

Daily Totals: 1,201 calories, 79 g protein, 143 g carbohydrates, 33 g fiber, 39 g fat, 6 g saturated fat, 1,345 mg sodium

To make it 1,500 calories: Increase Maple Granola to 1/3 cup at breakfast, increase to 10 walnut halves at A.M. snack, and add ¼ cup unsalted dry-roasted almonds to P.M. snack.

To make it 2,000 calories: Increase Maple Granola to 1/3 cup at breakfast and add 1 slice whole-wheat toast with 1½ Tbsp. almond butter, increase to 12 walnut halves at A.M. snack, add 1 serving Everything Bagel Avocado Toast to lunch, add ¼ cup unsalted dry-roasted almonds to P.M. snack, and add ½ an avocado at dinner.

Day 7

Breakfast (255 calories)

- 1 serving Strawberry-Pineapple Smoothie

A.M. Snack (30 calories)

- 1 plum

Lunch (304 calories)

- 1 serving Green Goddess Salad with Chickpeas

P.M. Snack (206 calories)

- ¼ cup unsalted dry-roasted almonds

Dinner (405 calories)

- 1 serving Sweet & Sour Chicken
- 2 cups mixed greens

- 1 Tbsp. Citrus Vinaigrette

Daily Totals: 1,201 calories, 66 g protein, 136 g carbohydrates, 33 g fiber, 51 g fat, 6 g saturated fat, 1,361 mg sodium

To make it 1,500 calories: Add 1 banana to breakfast and 15 walnut halves to A.M. snack.

To make it 2,000 calories: Add 1 slice whole-wheat toast with 1½ Tbsp. almond butter to breakfast, add ¼ cup unsalted dry-roasted almonds to A.M. snack, add 1 serving Everything Bagel Avocado Toast to lunch, and add 2 servings Vinegary Coleslaw to dinner.

Shrimp-&-Grits-Stuffed Peppers

Shrimp and grits are stuffed inside bell peppers and baked in this healthy stuffed peppers recipe. Add the optional hot sauce if you want to give the filling some kick. Look for bell peppers--use any color--

with even bottoms, so that they stand upright on their own when they're cooked.

Ingredients

- 1 ½ cups water
- 1 cup low-sodium chicken broth
- ¾ cup quick grits (not instant)
- ½ teaspoon ground pepper, divided
- ¾ cup shredded extra-sharp Cheddar cheese
- ½ teaspoon hot sauce, such as Tabasco (optional)
- 4 large bell peppers
- 1 pound peeled and deveined large shrimp (16-20 count), chopped
- 1 bunch scallions, trimmed and sliced
- 1 tablespoon extra-virgin olive oil
- ½ teaspoon garlic powder
- ¼ teaspoon salt

Directions

Step 1

Preheat oven to 350 degrees F.

Step 2

Bring water and broth to a boil in a large saucepan over medium-high heat. Whisk in grits and 1/4 teaspoon pepper. Reduce heat to medium-low; cover and cook, stirring occasionally, until thickened, 5 to 7 minutes. Remove from heat and stir in cheese and hot sauce (if using). Cover to keep warm.

Step 3

Slice off stem ends of bell peppers and scoop out the seeds from the cavities. Place the peppers on one end of a large rimmed baking sheet; bake for 5 minutes.

Step 4

While, in a medium cup, mix shrimp, scallions, sugar, garlic powder , salt and the remaining 1/4 tea poon pepper. Switch to the empty side of the sheet of baking, spreading uniformly. Bake, stir the shrimp mixture once, for about 10 minutes, until the peppers are softened and the shrimp just cooked through. Remove from the frying pan. Stir the shrimp mixture into the grits and then split the mixture between the 4 bell peppers. Bake for about 10 minutes, until the mixture is dry.

Nutrition Facts

Serving Size: 1 Pepper

Per Serving:

406 calories; 12.7 g total fat; 4.9 g saturated fat; 204 mg cholesterol; 454 mg sodium. 827 mg potassium; 40 g carbohydrates; 5.3 g fiber; 7 g sugar; 33.3 g protein; 5624 IU vitamin a iu; 214 mg vitamin c;

167 mcg folate; 259 mg calcium; 3 mg iron; 81 mg magnesium.

Mediterranean Broccoli Pasta Salad

Ingredients

- 8 ounces whole-wheat farfalle pasta
- 6 cups broccoli florets
- ½ cup chopped red bell pepper
- ¼ cup chopped red onion
- 2 tablespoons chopped fresh flat-leaf parsley
- 2 tablespoons chopped fresh basil
- ¾ cup mayonnaise
- ½ cup finely chopped sun-dried tomatoes in oil, drained
- 1 teaspoon lemon zest
- 1 teaspoon dried oregano
- ½ teaspoon salt
- ¼ teaspoon crushed red pepper

Directions

Step 1

Place a large ice-water bowl next to the stove. Take a big saucepan of water to boil. Cook pasta according to the instructions of the packet, adding broccoli to the water in the final 2 minutes of cooking time. Drain the broccoli and pasta; switch to the ice water; Drain fine. Add bell pepper, onion, parsley, and basil to a large bowl.

Step 2

Combine mayonnaise, sun-dried tomatoes, lemon zest, oregano, salt and crushed red pepper in a small bowl. Add to the pasta mixture; toss to coat.

Tips

To make ahead: Refrigerate in an airtight container for up to 1 day.

Nutrition Facts

Serving Size: About 1 Cup

Per Serving:

222 calories; 13.7 g total fat; 2.1 g saturated fat; 7 mg cholesterol; 250 mg sodium. 312 mg potassium; 21.9 g carbohydrates; 3.6 g fiber; 1 g sugar; 5.2 g protein; 1705 IU vitamin a iu; 57 mg vitamin c; 52 mcg folate; 40 mg calcium; 2 mg iron; 50 mg magnesium;

Exchanges:

2 1/2 Fat, 1 Starch, 1 Vegetable

7-Day DASH Diet Menu

Day 1

Breakfast (266 calories)

Egg Toast with Salsa

- 1 slice whole-wheat bread, toasted
- 1 egg, cooked in 1/4 tsp. olive oil
- Pinch each of salt and pepper
- 2 Tbsp. pico de gallo or salsa

Top bread with the egg, salt, pepper and pico de gallo.

- 1 medium banana

A.M. Snack (102 calories)

- 1 pear, sliced topped with cinnamon

Lunch (325 calories)

- 1 serving Veggie-Hummus Sandwich

P.M. Snack (48 calories)

- 3/4 cup raspberries

Dinner (450 calories)

- 1 serving Lemon-Herb Salmon with Caponata & Farro

Daily Totals: 1,192 calories, 60 g protein, 161 g carbohydrates, 37 g fiber, 40 g fat, 1,438 mg sodium

Day 2

Breakfast (258 calories)

Fig & Honey Yogurt

- 2/3 cup nonfat plain Greek yogurt

- 5 dried figs, chopped

- 2 tsp. chia seeds

- 1 1/2 tsp. honey

Top yogurt with figs, chia seeds and honey.

A.M. Snack (52 calories)

- 1/2 cup grapes

Lunch (350 calories)

White Bean & Avocado Salad

- 2 cups mixed greens

- 3/4 cup chopped veggies, such as cucumber and cherry tomatoes

- 1/3 cup canned white beans, rinsed

- 1/2 avocado, diced

- 2 Tbsp. All-Purpose Vinaigrette

Top salad greens with veggies, beans, avocado and vinaigrette. Toss to combine.

P.M. Snack (35 calories)

- 1 clementine

Dinner (489 calories)

- 1 serving Curried Cauliflower Steaks with Red Rice & Tzatziki

- 1 serving Chocolate & Nut Butter Bites, to enjoy after dinner

Daily Totals: 1,184 calories, 41 g protein, 155 g carbohydrates, 30 g fiber, 53 g fat, 818 mg sodium

Day 3

Breakfast (266 calories)

- 1 serving Peanut-Butter Cinnamon Toast

A.M. Snack (64 calories)

- 1 cup raspberries

Lunch (342 calories)

- 1 serving Salmon Pita Sandwich (save the other half of the pita for lunch on Day 5)

- 1 cup grapes

P.M. Snack (102 calories)

- 1 medium pear, sliced topped with cinnamon

Dinner (437 calories)

- 1 serving Mediterranean Chicken with Orzo Salad

- 1 clementine, to enjoy after dinner

Daily Totals: 1,212 calories, 69 g protein, 164 g carbohydrates, 30 g fiber, 35 g fat, 1,234 mg sodium

Day 4

Breakfast (251 calories)

Yogurt with Nuts & Raspberries

- 1 cup nonfat plain Greek yogurt

- 1/2 cup raspberries
- 5 walnuts, chopped
- 1 tsp. honey

Top yogurt with raspberries, walnuts and honey.

A.M. Snack 951 calories)

- 1 medium apple, sliced sprinkled with cinnamon

Lunch (332 calories)

- 1 serving White Bean & Avocado Toast
- 1 1/2 cups mixed greens
- 1/2 cup cucumber slices
- 2 Tbsp. grated carrot
- 1 Tbsp. All-Purpose Vinaigrette

Top salad greens with cucumber, carrot and vinaigrette. Toss to combine.

P.M. Snack (30 calories)

- 1 medium plum

Dinner (472 calories)

- 1 serving Stuffed Sweet Potato with Hummus Dressing

Daily Totals: 1,181 calories, 58 g protein, 176 g carbohydrates, 46 g fiber, 36 g fat, 976 mg sodium

Day 5

Breakfast (266 calories)

- 1 serving Peanut-Butter Cinnamon Toast

A.M. Snack (70 calories)

- 2 clementines

Lunch (332 calories)

Green Salad with Pita Bread & Hummus

- 2 cups mixed greens

- 1/4 cup grated carrot

- 1/2 cup sliced cucumber

- 2 Tbsp. All-Purpose Vinaigrette

- 1/2 large whole-wheat pita round

- 1/4 cup hummus

Top greens with carrot, cucumber and vinaigrette. Serve with pita bread and hummus

- 1 medium plum

P.M. Snack (104 calories)

- 1 cup grapes

Dinner (412 calories)

- 1 1/2 cups Chicken Chili with Sweet Potatoes

- 1/4 avocado, diced

- 1 Tbsp. nonfat plain Greek yogurt

Top chili with avocado and yogurt.

Meal-Prep Tip: Save 1 1/2 cups of the chili for lunch on Day 7.

Daily Totals: 1,184 calories, 50 g protein, 166 g carbohydrates, 31 g fiber, 42 g fat, 1,322 mg sodium

Day 6

Breakfast (258 calories)

Fig & Honey Yogurt

- 2/3 cup nonfat plain Greek yogurt
- 5 dried figs, chopped
- 2 tsp. chia seeds
- 1 1/2 tsp. honey

Top yogurt with figs, chia seeds and honey.

A.M. Snack (64 calories)

- 1 cup raspberries

Lunch (342 calories)

Turkey & Pear Pita Melt

- 1/2 large whole-wheat pita round (save the other half of the pita for a snack on Day 7)

- 3 1/2 oz. low-sodium deli turkey

- 1 medium pear, sliced

- 1 Tbsp. shredded Cheddar cheese

- 1 cup mixed greens

Stuff pita pocket with turkey, half of the pear slices and cheese. Toast in a toaster oven until the cheese starts to melt. Add greens to the pita just before eating. Serve the remaining pear slices on the side.

P.M. Snack (83 calories)

- 1 medium plum

- 4 walnuts halves

Dinner (469 calories)

- 1 serving Lemon-Garlic Shrimp over Orzo with Zucchini

- 1 clementine plus 1 serving Chocolate & Nut Butter Bites, to enjoy after dinner

Daily Totals: 1,216 calories, 80 g protein, 162 g carbohydrates, 30 g fiber, 31 g fat, 1,290 mg sodium

Day 7

Breakfast (266 calories)

Egg Toast with Salsa

- 1 slice whole-wheat bread, toasted

- 1 egg, cooked in 1/4 tsp. olive oil

- Pinch each of salt and pepper

- 2 Tbsp. pico de gallo or salsa

Top bread with egg, salt, pepper and pico de gallo.

- 1 medium banana

A.M. Snack (136 calories)

- 1/2 large whole-wheat pita round, toasted

- 2 Tbsp. hummus

Lunch (324 calories)

- 1 1/2 cups Chicken Chili with Sweet Potatoes

P.M. Snack (32 calories)

- 1/2 cup raspberries

Dinner (448 calories)

- 1 1/3 cups Creamy Fettuccine with Brussels Sprouts & Mushrooms

- 1/2 ounce dark chocolate, to enjoy after dinner

Daily Totals: 1,205 calories, 62 g protein, 171 g carbohydrates, 30 g fiber, 36 g fat, 1,754 mg sodium

7-Day Mediterranean Meal Plan

Day 1

Breakfast (324 calories)

- 1 serving Rainbow Frittata
- 1 medium banana

A.M. Snack (123 calories)

- 1 medium orange
- 8 unsalted almonds

Lunch (374 calories)

- 1 serving Green Salad with Pita Bread & Hummus

P.M. Snack (126 calories)

- 1 cup raspberries

- 1/2 cup whole-milk Greek yogurt

- 1 Tbsp. chia seeds

Dinner (442 calories)

- 1 serving Dijon Salmon with Green Bean Pilaf

Daily Totals: 1,501 calories, 79 g protein, 151 g carbohydrates, 37 g fiber, 71 g fat, 1,640 mg sodium

Day 2

Breakfast (365 calories)

- 1 serving Muesli with Raspberries

- 1 hard-boiled egg

A.M. Snack (92 calories)

- 1 plum

- 8 unsalted almonds

Lunch (337 calories)

- 1 serving Brussels Sprouts Salad with Crispy Chickpeas

P.M. Snack (102 calories)

- 2 Tbsp. hummus

- 2 medium carrots

Dinner (593 calories)

- 1 serving Linguine with Creamy Mushroom Sauce

- 1 serving Basic Green Salad with Vinaigrette

Daily Totals: 1,489 calories, 56 g protein, 171 g carbohydrates, 43 g fiber, 70 g fat, 1,310 mg sodium

Day 3

Breakfast (357 calories)

- 1 serving Fig & Ricotta Toast

- 1 medium banana

A.M. Snack (122 calories)

- 2 plums

- 8 unsalted almonds

Lunch (431 calories)

- 1 serving Brussels Sprouts Salad with Crispy Chickpeas

- 1 medium apple

P.M. Snack (177 calories)

- 1 cup raspberries

- 1/4 cup whole-milk Greek yogurt

- 1 Tbsp. chia seeds

Dinner (429 calories)

- 1 serving Cod in Tomato Cream Sauce

- 1 cup Basic Quinoa

Daily Totals: 1,517 calories, 65 g protein, 197 g carbohydrates, 45 g fiber, 56 g fat, 1,134 mg sodium

Day 4

Breakfast (368 calories)

- 1 serving Creamy Blueberry-Pecan Overnight Oats

- 1 hard-boiled egg

A.M. Snack (176 calories)

- 1 medium orange

- 1 ounce cheddar cheese

Lunch (337 calories)

- 1 serving Brussels Sprouts Salad with Crispy Chickpeas

Afternoon Snack (122 calories)

- 2 plums

- 8 unsalted almonds

Dinner (477 calories)

- 1 serving Mediterranean Chickpea Quinoa Bowl

Daily Totals: 1,481 calories, 51 g protein, 163 g carbohydrates, 33 g fiber, 74 g fat, 1,417 mg sodium

Day 5

Breakfast (365 calories)

- 1 serving Muesli with Raspberries
- 1 hard-boiled egg

A.M. Snack (31 calories)

- 1 plum

Lunch (431 calories)

- 1 serving Brussels Sprouts Salad with Crispy Chickpeas

- 1 medium apple

P.M. Snack (176 calories)

- 1 medium orange

- 1 ounce cheddar cheese

Dinner (491 calories)

- 2 generous cups Chicken & White Bean Soup

- 1-inch thick slice baguette

Meal-Prep Tip: Save 1 1/2 cups of the Chicken & White Bean Soup to have for lunch on Day 6.

Daily Totals: 1,493 calories, 96 g protein, 180 g carbohydrates, 42 g fiber, 51 g fat, 1,330 mg sodium

Day 6

Breakfast (368 calories)

- 1 serving Creamy Blueberry-Pecan Overnight Oats

- 1 hard-boiled egg

A.M. Snack (62 calories)

- 1 medium orange

Lunch (342 calories)

- 1 1/2 cups Chicken & White Bean Soup

- 1 medium apple

P.M. Snack (129 calories)

- 3 Tbsp. hummus

- 2 medium carrots

Dinner (491 calories)

- 1 serving Eggs in Tomato Sauce with Chickpeas & Spinach

- 1 large whole wheat pita

Daily Totals: 1,515 calories, 78 g protein, 188 g carbohydrates, 35 g fiber, 44 g fat, 1,702 mg sodium

Day 7

Breakfast (357 calories)

- 1 serving Fig & Ricotta Toast

- 1 medium banana

A.M. Snack (145 calories)

- 1/2 cup raspberries

- 1/4 cup whole-milk Greek Yogurt

- 1 Tbsp. chia seeds

Lunch (374 calories)

- 1 serving Green Salad with Pita Bread & Hummus

P.M. Snack (102 calories)

- 2 Tbsp. hummus

- 2 medium carrots

Dinner (397 calories)

- 1 serving Slow-Cooker Mediterranean Chicken & Orzo

- 1-inch thick slice baguette

Evening Snack (125 calories)

- 5 fluid ounces red wine

Daily Totals: 1,499 calories, 72 g protein, 201 g carbohydrates, 39 g fiber, 39 g fat, 1,935 mg sodium.

www.ingramcontent.com/pod-product-compliance
Lightning Source LLC
Chambersburg PA
CBHW050247220526
45465CB00002B/579